The Plant Prescription

Harnessing Nature's Healing Power for Physical Well-being

Aspen Sunhaven

DISCLAIMER

This book is intended for informational and entertainment purposes only. It is not a substitute for professional medical advice, diagnosis, or treatment. Always seek the advice of your physician or other qualified health provider with any questions you may have regarding a medical condition.

Table of Contents

DISCLAIMER...iii

Table of Contents...iv

Acknowledgments..1

Introduction: The Healing Power of Plants.............................2

Rediscovering Nature's Pharmacy..2

Chapter 1: The Science of Plant-Based Healing......................5

Chapter 2: Ancient Traditions, Modern Solutions.................11

Chapter 3: Incorporating Plant Remedies Into Daily Life.........16

Chapter 4: Healing Through Nature's Aromas........................19

Chapter 5: Plants and Mental Health: Beyond Physical Healing..25

Chapter 6: The Healing Power of Herbal Teas and Tinctures.....31

Chapter 7: Detoxing Your Body with Plants............................37

Chapter 8: Strengthening Immunity with Plant Power............43

Chapter 9: Healing Skin and Body with Natural Remedies..........49

Chapter 10: The Future of Plant-Based Medicine....................55

Chapter 11: Healing Skin and Body with Natural Remedies........61

Chapter 12: Reflections..69

Acknowledgments

Writing "The Plant Prescription" has been a journey of deep gratitude and discovery, a testament to the enduring wisdom of nature and its profound ability to heal and nourish.

I extend my heartfelt thanks to the plants themselves – for their resilience, their generosity, and their quiet lessons in well-being.

To my family and friends, thank you for your unwavering love and support. Your encouragement has been a balm for my soul, fueling my passion for sharing the healing power of plants.

And to you, dear reader, thank you for embarking on this journey with me. May the knowledge within these pages empower you to embrace nature's pharmacy and cultivate a life of vibrant health and vitality.

With love and gratitude,

Aspen Sunhaven

Introduction: The Healing Power of Plants Rediscovering Nature's Pharmacy

From the lush rainforests of the Amazon to the sun-kissed meadows of Provence, the natural world teems with a vibrant tapestry of plants, each holding within its leaves, roots, and blossoms a unique potential for healing and well-being. For centuries, humans have turned to these botanical wonders for remedies, harnessing their power to soothe ailments, restore balance, and promote vitality. In an age where modern medicine often dominates our approach to health, there's a growing yearning to reconnect with the wisdom of nature and rediscover the healing potential of plants.

In "The Plant Prescription," we embark on a journey to explore this timeless connection, delving into the science behind plant-based healing, uncovering the secrets of ancient traditions, and discovering practical ways to incorporate natural remedies into our modern lives. We'll journey through the vibrant world of botanicals, learning about their unique properties and how they can support our physical health in a gentle yet powerful way.

Natural Remedies: A Growing Movement

In recent years, there's been a resurgence of interest in natural remedies and plant-based healing. As we become increasingly aware of the potential side effects of synthetic drugs and the limitations of conventional medicine, many of us are seeking gentler, more holistic approaches to health and wellness. We're drawn to the wisdom of our ancestors, who relied on plants for their medicinal needs, and we're inspired by the growing body of scientific evidence that supports the efficacy of many traditional remedies.

From herbal teas and tinctures to aromatherapy and topical applications, plant-based remedies offer a wealth of options for supporting our physical well-being. They can help us to boost our immunity, reduce inflammation, improve digestion, promote restful sleep, and support cardiovascular health, among other benefits. And perhaps most importantly, they can empower us to take an active role in our own health, connecting us to the natural world and its inherent healing potential.

Bridging Modern Medicine with Nature's Wisdom

While modern medicine has undoubtedly made remarkable advances in treating and preventing diseases, it's not always the only or the best answer. The complexity of the human body and the interconnectedness of our physical, emotional, and spiritual well-being often require a more holistic approach to health.

Plant-based remedies, rooted in centuries of traditional use and supported by modern scientific research, offer a bridge between ancient wisdom and contemporary healthcare. They provide us with gentle yet effective tools for supporting our bodies' natural healing processes and promoting optimal well-being.

In the following chapters, we'll explore the science of plant-based healing, delve into the rich tapestry of ancient herbal traditions, and discover practical ways to incorporate natural remedies into our daily lives. We'll learn how to create a natural first-aid kit, brew healing teas and tinctures, and harness the power of aromatherapy to support our physical health.

We'll also journey beyond the physical realm, exploring the profound connection between plants and mental health, and discovering how nature's remedies can soothe our minds and nurture our emotional well-being.

As we embark on this exploration, let's approach the world of plant-based healing with an open mind and a curious heart. Let's embrace the wisdom of our ancestors, the insights of modern science, and the gentle power of plants to guide us on a path to lifelong wellness.

With this foundation laid, let's begin our journey into the world of botanical healing by exploring the scientific foundations of plant-based medicine

Chapter 1: The Science of Plant-Based Healing

How Plants Influence Our Bodies at a Cellular Level

Throughout history, humans have turned to the natural world for healing, relying on plants to soothe ailments, prevent disease, and promote wellness. From lush rainforests to herbal gardens, plants have served as humanity's pharmacy, offering remedies for a wide variety of conditions. Today, science is uncovering the powerful ways plants impact our bodies, providing concrete evidence of their ability to heal on a cellular level. This chapter dives deep into the mechanisms of plant-based healing, showing how these natural wonders interact with our biology to support physical and emotional well-being.

The Cellular Symphony: How Plants Heal from Within

At the core of our health are trillions of cells, each functioning like tiny engines, fueling our bodies and maintaining homeostasis. Just like a city that requires balanced communication, energy, and protection, our cells need nutrients, antioxidants, and protection from environmental damage. When these systems fail, disease and dysfunction can follow.

Plants, rich in bioactive compounds called phytonutrients, can serve as the conductors of this cellular symphony. These compounds—responsible for giving plants their vibrant colors, flavors, and smells—also possess powerful medicinal properties. Phytonutrients interact with our cells in myriad ways, from modulating gene expression to promoting the repair of damaged tissues.

For instance, flavonoids—found in fruits like blueberries—have been shown to enhance brain function by increasing blood flow to key areas, improving memory and cognition. Carotenoids, abundant in carrots and sweet potatoes, support eye health by protecting the retina from oxidative damage. Alkaloids like those found in green tea help to reduce inflammation and enhance cellular communication.

These compounds work not only to prevent disease but also to restore balance when things go wrong. This idea of cellular homeostasis is key to understanding how plant-based healing works—plants don't just treat symptoms; they address the root causes of illness by working on a cellular level.

Phytonutrients: The Body's Best Ally

Plants have evolved an impressive array of defense mechanisms to protect themselves from environmental threats. In the process, they've developed compounds that can do the same for us. Phytonutrients, though not essential for survival like vitamins and minerals, are crucial for optimal health. They offer protection against a wide range of chronic conditions, including heart disease, cancer, and neurodegenerative diseases.

Antioxidants:

Antioxidants like flavonoids and polyphenols neutralize harmful free radicals—unstable molecules that can damage cells and accelerate aging. Found in colorful fruits and vegetables, antioxidants act as shields, protecting our cells from oxidative stress. Studies have shown that regular consumption of antioxidant-rich foods can reduce the risk of cardiovascular disease, slow down the aging process, and even improve cognitive function.

Anti-Inflammatory Agents:

Chronic inflammation is the root cause of many modern ailments, from arthritis to heart disease. Plants like turmeric contain curcumin, a potent anti-inflammatory compound that can reduce inflammation at the molecular level. Ginger, with its active compound gingerol, has also been shown to reduce inflammation, particularly in conditions like osteoarthritis and muscle pain.

Immune Boosters:

Certain plants have immune-modulating effects, helping to enhance the body's defense mechanisms. Echinacea, for instance, stimulates the production of white blood cells, boosting the body's ability to fight off infections. Garlic, with its active compound allicin, is another potent immune booster, known for its antibacterial, antiviral, and antifungal properties.

Plant-Based Healing in Practice: Common Medicinal Plants

The world of medicinal plants is vast, but some have stood out for their proven efficacy in supporting health and well-being. Here's a closer look at a few commonly used medicinal plants and their healing properties:

Turmeric (Curcuma longa):

Turmeric's active compound, curcumin, has been widely studied for its powerful anti-inflammatory and antioxidant effects. It is particularly effective in treating chronic inflammation, such as in conditions like arthritis and inflammatory bowel disease. Studies suggest that curcumin may also play a role in preventing Alzheimer's disease by reducing amyloid plaque buildup in the brain.

Ginger (Zingiber officinale):

Ginger has been used for centuries to alleviate nausea and improve digestion. Its anti-inflammatory properties also make it effective in treating osteoarthritis and muscle soreness. Recent research indicates that ginger may also have anticancer properties, particularly in suppressing the growth of certain types of cancer cells.

Garlic (Allium sativum):

Garlic is one of the most well-researched medicinal plants. Its active compound, allicin, offers a range of health benefits, including reducing blood pressure, lowering cholesterol, and improving immune function. Garlic is also known for its cardiovascular benefits, with studies showing that it can reduce the risk of heart disease by improving blood flow and reducing blood clot formation.

Echinacea (Echinacea purpurea):

Echinacea is best known for its immune-boosting properties. Often taken as a preventative remedy for colds and flu, it works by stimulating the activity of white blood cells. Some studies suggest that echinacea can shorten the duration of colds and reduce the severity of symptoms.

Plants and Cellular Communication: Fine-Tuning the Body

One of the most remarkable aspects of plant-based healing is how plants can influence cellular communication within the body. Cells rely on complex signaling pathways to maintain homeostasis and coordinate the body's response to various challenges. Certain plants, through their phytonutrients, can enhance or modulate these pathways.

Adaptogens, such as ashwagandha and rhodiola, help the body adapt to stress by balancing hormones and reducing the harmful effects of chronic stress on the body. They work by modulating the stress-response system, allowing the body to maintain homeostasis even in the face of external pressures. These plants are particularly beneficial in modern life, where chronic stress is a major contributor to illness.

Embracing Plant-Based Healing for a Healthier Future

The science of plant-based healing is a testament to the power of nature. By understanding how plants influence our bodies at the cellular level, we can harness their potential to prevent disease, support recovery, and promote overall well-being. As we continue to explore the world of medicinal plants, it's important to remember that the healing power of nature is not a quick fix but a long-term, sustainable approach to health.

Through mindful consumption of plant-based remedies, we can cultivate a healthier, more balanced life, one that honors the wisdom of nature and our deep connection to the world around us. As you incorporate these green allies into your wellness routine, know that you are participating in a timeless tradition of healing, one that has been practiced for millennia and continues to offer hope for a vibrant, healthy future.

Chapter 2: Ancient Traditions, Modern Solutions

Whispers from the Past, Echoes in the Present

Imagine standing in a sunlit meadow, where a sea of wildflowers sways gently in the breeze. Picture the sunlight streaming through the branches of a majestic forest, casting a soft, golden glow on the earth below. Breathe in the intoxicating scent of jasmine in full bloom or the rich, earthy aroma of moss-covered tree roots. Nature, in all its splendor, is an endless source of beauty, offering a world of inspiration for those willing to look. Its vibrant colors, intricate textures, and subtle forms are waiting to ignite your imagination and stir your creative spirit.

In this chapter, we'll explore the extraordinary world of botanical beauty, discovering how plants can serve as your muse. From the brilliant colors of a blooming garden to the intricate designs of leaves and petals, we'll uncover how the beauty of the plant kingdom can spark creativity, evoke emotions, and lead you on a path of artistic expression.

A Kaleidoscope of Colors: Nature's Emotional Palette

The natural world is a living canvas, painted with shifting hues that change with each season. From the fiery oranges and reds of autumn to the soft pinks and greens of spring, every color tells a story, evokes a feeling, and invites us to explore it.

The Emotional Power of Color: Colors have a unique ability to affect our emotions and perceptions. Warm tones like red, orange, and yellow are energizing and invigorating, while cool shades of blue, green, and purple inspire calm and tranquility. By paying attention to the colors found in nature, you can draw inspiration and infuse emotional depth into your work.

Nature's Color Wheel in Action: I once walked through a meadow of wildflowers in the Sierra Nevada mountains. The bright purples, oranges, and reds of lupines, poppies, and Indian paintbrush created a vivid masterpiece around me. As I took in the vibrant scene, I felt my heart lift, my mind buzz with new ideas, and my senses awaken to the beauty around me.

Bringing Nature's Colors into Your Art: Whether you are painting, writing, or composing music, there are endless ways to bring the colors of nature into your art. You might use bold strokes of paint to mimic the energy of a sunset or write a poem that captures the quiet beauty of a dewy morning. However you choose to express yourself, the colors of the natural world will infuse your art with vibrancy and emotion.

Textures That Tantalize: The Tactile Symphony of Nature

Nature is filled with textures that draw us in and invite us to engage our senses. From the smoothness of a flower petal to the rough bark of a tree, these textures offer a tactile experience that can evoke memories, emotions, and ideas.

The Language of Texture: Texture adds depth and dimension to artistic work, helping create a multi-sensory experience. By incorporating nature's textures into your creations, you can connect with your audience on a more intimate level, evoking the feel of the natural world through your medium.

Nature's Textured Tapestry: I'm constantly fascinated by the textures in my own garden. The velvety softness of lamb's ears, the prickly spines of cacti, and the delicate veins on maple leaves all inspire me. Take a moment to explore the textures around you— whether it's the smooth surface of a river stone or the grain of wood—and let them guide your creativity.

Translating Texture Into Your Work: Artists working with paint, clay, fabric, or words can use texture to bring their work to life. You might experiment with rough, bold brushstrokes or choose smooth, flowing ones to evoke softness. Writers can describe textures to bring their words to life, while musicians can use rhythm to convey the feel of different surfaces. Allow the textures of nature to inspire and enhance your artistic expression.

Forms That Fascinate: The Geometry of Nature

Nature is filled with beautiful, complex designs that can serve as inspiration for creative work. From the spiral arrangement of sunflower seeds to the perfect symmetry of flowers, the geometry of the natural world is a marvel of design and form.

The Language of Form: Forms convey movement, balance, and harmony in art, giving structure to creative ideas. By observing the forms of nature—whether in the curves of a vine or the geometric shapes of a pinecone—you can tap into a source of beauty that resonates deeply with viewers.

Exploring Nature's Geometric Playground: Take a closer look at the plants around you. Notice how the leaves of a fern uncurl in a perfect spiral or how the branches of a tree extend outward in an intricate, balanced pattern. These forms offer a sense of wonder, reminding us that nature is a master of design.

Bringing Nature's Forms into Your Art: Sculptors, writers, architects, and even musicians can translate nature's forms into their work. Try incorporating the symmetry of a flower into your designs or use the spiral shape of a shell as inspiration for a poem. Experiment with how these shapes and structures can influence your artistic vision.

Fragrances That Evoke: Nature's Aromatic Symphony

The scents of the natural world have the power to transport us, stir emotions, and evoke memories. The sweet fragrance of jasmine, the sharp scent of pine needles, or the earthy aroma of soil can all inspire us to create.

The Power of Scent: Scents can evoke a wide range of emotions, from joy to nostalgia. They can also transport us to different places, from a peaceful garden to a bustling spice market. By incorporating scents into your creative process, you can add an extra layer of depth to your work.

Exploring Nature's Aromas: Take a moment to inhale the fragrances around you. Notice the delicate perfume of a blooming rose or the crisp smell of fallen leaves. Let these aromas spark your creativity and guide your expression.

Capturing Fragrance in Your Art: Although scent is difficult to capture directly in visual or auditory art, you can evoke it through imagery, texture, and atmosphere. You might also use essential oils or aromatic herbs to create a calming, inspiring environment while you work, allowing the fragrances of nature to influence your creations.

.

Chapter 3: Incorporating Plant Remedies Into Daily Life

Nature's Touch in Your Everyday

Imagine your medicine cabinet filled not with synthetic pills, but with nature's remedies—herbs, teas, and tinctures that have been used for generations to soothe, heal, and restore. Incorporating plant remedies into your daily routine can be a simple yet profound way to nurture your well-being, just as a garden nurtures life.

Plant-Based Supplements are one way to access the healing power of plants, offering concentrated doses of phytonutrients and other beneficial compounds. But with the vast array of supplements available, it's important to choose wisely. Look for supplements from reputable brands, those that use organic and sustainably sourced ingredients. Consulting with a healthcare professional before starting new supplements is always recommended, particularly if you have underlying health conditions.

When incorporating supplements, start slowly, allowing your body to adjust. Keep in mind that whole herbs often offer a more balanced approach than isolated compounds. For example, the whole turmeric root contains a synergy of compounds that work together more effectively than isolated curcumin alone.

Another essential way to integrate plant remedies is by creating a natural first-aid kit filled with nature's powerful healing tools. Imagine reaching for lavender oil to soothe a minor burn or peppermint oil to ease digestive discomfort. These simple remedies offer effective and gentle ways to address common health concerns.

Here are a few essentials to include in your natural first-aid kit:

Lavender essential oil for burns, insect bites, and headaches.

Arnica gel to soothe muscle soreness and bruises.

Chamomile tea bags promote relaxation and ease anxiety.

Aloe vera gel for sunburns and skin irritations.

Lastly, one of the most enjoyable ways to embrace plant remedies is through your diet. Fresh and dried herbs like basil, oregano, and parsley are easy to add to meals, boosting flavor while providing a nutritional punch. Herbal teas are another simple and effective way to enjoy the benefits of plants daily, offering both hydration and healing.

Incorporating plants into your daily life is about more than just health—it's about empowerment. By learning to use these remedies, you take an active role in your wellness, trusting in nature's ability to support you.

Chapter 4: Healing Through Nature's Aromas

Essential Oils and Their Impact on the Body

The scent of freshly cut herbs, the invigorating aroma of pine trees after rainfall, or the calming fragrance of lavender fields at sunset—these natural scents do more than just please the senses. They also carry profound healing properties that affect both the mind and body. Aromatherapy, the practice of using essential oils derived from plants, taps into these benefits to support physical health and emotional well-being. In this chapter, we'll explore the power of essential oils, how they interact with the body, and ways to create a healing atmosphere with nature's scents.

The Science Behind Aromatherapy

Essential oils are highly concentrated extracts from plants, capturing the unique essence and medicinal properties of the plant in a small vial of oil. Through processes like distillation or cold pressing, the volatile compounds within the plants are released, creating oils that can influence physical and mental health.

The olfactory system, responsible for our sense of smell, plays a key role in aromatherapy's effects. When you inhale the scent of an essential oil, the molecules travel through the nasal passages to the olfactory bulb, which sends signals directly to the brain's limbic system—an area that influences emotions, memories, and survival instincts. This direct connection explains why certain smells can evoke strong memories or emotions and why aromatherapy is effective for stress relief, relaxation, and mood enhancement.

But beyond the emotional impact, essential oils also have physical effects. Many oils contain antimicrobial, anti-inflammatory, and immune-boosting properties, making them valuable tools in holistic healing.

Creating a Healing Atmosphere with Plants

Using essential oils is one of the most accessible ways to bring nature's aromas into your living space and create a soothing, healing environment. Diffusing oils in a room can fill the air with calming, invigorating, or balancing scents, depending on the oil you choose.

Lavender Oil: Known for its calming properties, lavender is one of the most popular essential oils for relaxation. Diffuse it in the evening to create a tranquil atmosphere that promotes restful sleep or add a few drops to a warm bath for a soothing, spa-like experience.

Peppermint Oil: For an invigorating and energizing boost, peppermint oil is excellent for enhancing focus and clearing mental fog.

It's perfect for a home office or workspace where clarity and creativity are needed.

Eucalyptus Oil: This oil is commonly used to support respiratory health. It's refreshing, minty scent helps to open airways, making it a great addition to a diffuser during cold and flu season or after a workout to ease breathing.

Frankincense Oil: Often referred to as the "king of essential oils," frankincense has been used for centuries in spiritual and religious practices. Its earthy aroma can promote feelings of peace and grounding, making it ideal for meditation or mindfulness sessions.

By thoughtfully incorporating essential oils into your daily life, you can create spaces that nurture your well-being, providing a natural escape from the stresses of modern life.

How Scents Affect Physical Well-being

Essential oils work not only on an emotional level but also have tangible effects on the body. For centuries, they've been used as remedies for various physical ailments, from skin irritations to digestive issues. Here are a few common ways that essential oils can impact physical well-being:

Pain Relief: Oils like eucalyptus, rosemary, and peppermint are frequently used to ease muscle tension, reduce pain, and alleviate headaches. A few drops can be added to a carrier oil like coconut oil and applied to sore muscles or temples for immediate relief.

Immune Support: Certain essential oils, such as tea tree and oregano, have potent antimicrobial properties that can help strengthen the body's defenses. By diffusing these oils or adding them to cleaning solutions, you can support your immune system and keep your environment fresh and healthy.

Skin Healing: Oils like tea tree, lavender, and chamomile can be applied to cuts, scrapes, or minor burns to promote faster healing and reduce the risk of infection. Dilute these oils with a carrier oil before applying to the skin to avoid irritation.

Essential oils are highly concentrated, so it's important to use them mindfully. Diluting oils before topical application, using only a few drops in diffusers, and researching which oils are safe for specific conditions are essential steps to ensure safe and effective use.

Recipes for Daily Aromatherapy

Here are a few simple ways to incorporate essential oils into your daily routine for both physical and emotional support:

Relaxing Room Spray: Combine 10 drops of lavender oil, 5 drops of chamomile oil, and 5 drops of bergamot oil with 1 cup of distilled water. Pour the mixture into a spray bottle and mist your bedroom or living space for a calming effect.

Focus and Clarity Diffuser Blend: In a diffuser, add 5 drops of peppermint oil, 5 drops of rosemary oil, and 5 drops of lemon oil to boost focus and mental clarity during work or study sessions.

Immune-Boosting Hand Sanitizer: Mix 5 drops of tea tree oil and 5 drops of lemon oil with 1 tablespoon of aloe vera gel and 1 tablespoon of witch hazel. Use as a natural hand sanitizer to keep germs at bay while nourishing the skin.

Headache Relief Roll-On: In a 10ml roller bottle, combine 10 drops of peppermint oil, 5 drops of eucalyptus oil, and 5 drops of lavender oil with a carrier oil like sweet almond or jojoba oil. Apply to the temples, back of the neck, and wrists to ease tension headaches.

By embracing the art of aromatherapy, you can transform your home into a sanctuary of well-being. With a few drops of essential oil, you can shift the energy of a space, calm your mind, soothe your body, and invite the healing power of plants into your life. Whether you're seeking relaxation, pain relief, or emotional balance, essential oils offer a simple yet profound way to support your holistic health.

Chapter 5: Plants and Mental Health: Beyond Physical Healing

The Holistic Approach to Emotional Well-being

When we think of plants, we often focus on their physical healing properties—their ability to ease pain, reduce inflammation, or support immunity. However, plants also offer profound benefits for our mental health, acting as natural allies in our quest for emotional balance and well-being. In this chapter, we'll explore the holistic approach that plants provide, focusing on how they can soothe the mind, promote relaxation, and help alleviate symptoms of anxiety, depression, and insomnia.

The Mind-Body Connection: Healing on Multiple Levels

The human body is not simply a collection of physical components. Emotional and mental well-being are deeply intertwined with physical health, creating an inseparable connection between mind and body. Plants have long been used in holistic healing traditions to address both mental and physical ailments simultaneously. Whether it's through the calming scent of lavender or the uplifting effects of lemon balm, plants can offer emotional support while also enhancing overall health.

The idea of treating emotional distress through plants dates back thousands of years. Ancient healing traditions, from Ayurveda to Traditional Chinese Medicine, have recognized the importance of addressing mental health as part of a holistic treatment. Today, modern research continues to uncover the benefits of plant-based remedies for mental well-being.

Herbs and Plants for Anxiety, Depression, and Better Sleep

Anxiety, depression, and sleep disturbances are among the most common mental health challenges in today's fast-paced world. While conventional treatments like therapy and medication play important roles, many people are turning to natural remedies to complement their mental health care. Here are a few plant-based options that can help support mental and emotional balance:

Lavender (Lavandula angustifolia): Widely known for its calming effects, lavender can help reduce symptoms of anxiety and stress. Its soothing aroma has been shown to promote relaxation and improve sleep quality. Drinking lavender tea or using lavender essential oil in a diffuser before bed can be particularly helpful for those struggling with insomnia.

Ashwagandha (Withania somnifera): This adaptogenic herb has been used in Ayurvedic medicine for centuries to help the body adapt to stress. Ashwagandha has been shown to reduce anxiety levels, improve mood, and even enhance cognitive function, making it a powerful tool for those managing chronic stress and anxiety disorders.

St. John's Wort (Hypericum perforatum): Commonly used to treat mild to moderate depression, St. John's Wort is believed to work by increasing levels of serotonin, a neurotransmitter associated with mood regulation. While it has been shown to be effective for some individuals, it is important to consult with a healthcare provider before using St. John's Wort, as it can interact with certain medications.

Chamomile (Matricaria chamomilla): Chamomile is well known for its calming properties and is frequently used to promote relaxation and reduce anxiety. Chamomile tea is a popular bedtime drink for those seeking a peaceful night's sleep, and its gentle nature makes it suitable for people of all ages.

Lemon Balm (Melissa officinalis): Lemon balm has a mild sedative effect and is often used to ease anxiety, promote calmness, and improve mood. It can be enjoyed as a tea or used as an essential oil for relaxation.

These plants offer a natural way to manage emotional well-being, working gently yet effectively to bring balance to the mind and body.

Nourishing the Nervous System: How Plants Soothe the Mind

Our nervous system plays a key role in how we experience stress and manage our emotions. When the nervous system is overstimulated, it can lead to anxiety, restlessness, and difficulty sleeping. Plants can support the nervous system in several ways, helping to calm and nourish it.

Valerian Root (Valeriana officinalis): Often referred to as "nature's Valium," valerian root has been used for centuries to promote relaxation and improve sleep. It is known for its sedative properties, which help to calm an overactive mind and soothe the nervous system. Valerian can be taken as a supplement, in tea form, or as an extract.

Passionflower (Passiflora incarnata): This herb is often used as a natural remedy for anxiety and insomnia. It works by increasing levels of gamma-aminobutyric acid (GABA) in the brain, which helps to calm the nervous system and promote feelings of relaxation. Passionflower is commonly taken in tea or tincture form before bed.

Skullcap (Scutellaria lateriflora): Skullcap is another herb known for its ability to calm the nervous system and ease tension. It is particularly useful for individuals who experience muscle tightness or headaches due to stress. Skullcap can be enjoyed as a tea or in tincture form.

These plants work harmoniously with the body to support the nervous system, encouraging relaxation and reducing the physical symptoms of stress.

The Emotional and Physical Health Connection

When we care for our mental health, we are also caring for our physical health. Stress, anxiety, and depression can take a significant toll on the body, leading to a range of physical symptoms such as digestive issues, headaches, muscle tension, and weakened immunity. By addressing mental health concerns through plant-based remedies, we are not only nurturing our minds but also supporting our bodies.

For example, herbs like peppermint and ginger can soothe digestive discomfort that often accompanies anxiety, while lavender and chamomile can ease muscle tension and headaches caused by stress. The beauty of plant-based remedies lies in their ability to address both emotional and physical symptoms simultaneously, promoting holistic well-being.

Incorporating Plant Remedies into Your Routine

Integrating plant-based remedies into your daily life is a simple yet effective way to support mental health. Here are a few practical tips for incorporating these healing plants into your routine:

Herbal Teas: Start your day with a calming cup of herbal tea, such as chamomile or lemon balm, to set a peaceful tone. In the evening, unwind with a blend of lavender and valerian tea to promote relaxation and restful sleep.

Essential Oils: Use essential oils like lavender or bergamot in a diffuser to create a calming atmosphere in your home or workspace. You can also apply diluted essential oils to your wrists or temples for on-the-go relaxation.

Herbal Baths: Add a handful of dried herbs, such as lavender, chamomile, or rosemary, to your bathwater for a soothing and stress-relieving soak.

Natural Supplements: Consider taking herbal supplements like ashwagandha or valerian root to support your body's response to stress and promote emotional balance.

By incorporating these simple practices into your daily routine, you can harness the power of plants to support your mental health and well-being in a natural, gentle way.

Plants offer a wealth of natural remedies for mental health, helping us to find calm, balance, and peace in an increasingly stressful world. Whether you're looking to reduce anxiety, improve sleep, or simply enhance your emotional well-being, plants provide a holistic approach that nurtures both the mind and body. Through mindful use of these healing botanicals, we can cultivate a life of emotional resilience and mental clarity.

Chapter 6: The Healing Power of Herbal Teas and Tinctures

Nature's Potions for Wellness

Throughout history, herbal teas and tinctures have been cherished for their therapeutic properties, serving as time-tested remedies for a wide array of physical and emotional ailments. In this chapter, we explore the art and science behind these plant-based potions, delving into how they promote healing, support overall well-being, and can be seamlessly integrated into daily life.

Herbal Teas: Sipping on Nature's Healing Elixir

Herbal teas have been used for thousands of years as a gentle yet effective way to deliver the medicinal properties of plants. Unlike traditional teas made from Camellia sinensis (the tea plant), herbal teas are created by steeping a variety of herbs, leaves, flowers, seeds, or roots in hot water. The process extracts the plant's active compounds, releasing their therapeutic benefits into a soothing and flavorful beverage.

Each herb carries its own distinct medicinal properties, offering support for everything from digestion and immunity to stress relief and sleep enhancement.

Key Benefits of Herbal Teas:

Calming the Mind: Herbal teas like chamomile and lavender are well known for their calming properties, helping to reduce anxiety and promote relaxation. Sipping these teas before bed can help unwind the mind and body, preparing you for a peaceful night's sleep.

Digestive Support: Herbs like peppermint and ginger aid digestion by soothing the stomach, alleviating nausea, and reducing bloating. These teas are commonly consumed after meals to promote digestive comfort.

Boosting Immunity: Plants like echinacea and elderberry are often used in teas to strengthen the immune system, especially during cold and flu season. Drinking these teas regularly can help your body fend off infections and recover more quickly.

Herbal teas provide a simple, delicious, and effective way to incorporate the healing power of plants into your daily routine. By selecting the right herbs for your individual needs, you can create custom blends that support your physical and emotional health.

Tinctures: Concentrated Plant Power for Healing

Tinctures are potent liquid extracts made by soaking herbs in alcohol or vinegar to extract their medicinal compounds. Unlike herbal teas, tinctures are highly concentrated, making them an efficient way to harness the healing power of plants in small, easy-to-use doses. Tinctures are often taken by placing a few drops under the tongue or mixing them into water, tea, or juice.

Why Choose Tinctures?

Potency: Due to their concentrated nature, tinctures offer a higher potency of the active compounds found in plants, allowing for a more intense therapeutic effect.

Convenience: Tinctures are portable and easy to incorporate into daily life. Whether you're at home, at work, or on the go, you can carry a small bottle with you and take your daily dose as needed.

Long Shelf Life: Tinctures have a much longer shelf life than fresh herbs or teas, typically lasting several years when stored in a cool, dark place.

Common Tinctures and Their Uses:

Valerian Root: Known for its calming properties, valerian tincture is often used to alleviate stress, anxiety, and insomnia.

Echinacea: This immune-boosting tincture is widely used to prevent and treat colds and flu, helping the body fight off infections.

Milk Thistle: Popular for supporting liver health, milk thistle tincture aids in detoxification and promotes liver regeneration.

By incorporating tinctures into your wellness routine, you can enjoy a convenient and potent way to experience the medicinal benefits of plants.

Recipes for Common Ailments Using Herbal Teas and Tinctures

Herbal teas and tinctures can be easily customized to address specific health concerns. Below are a few simple recipes that showcase the healing potential of these plant-based remedies:

Relaxation and Sleep Support Tea

Ingredients:

1 tsp dried chamomile

1 tsp dried lavender

1 tsp lemon balm

1 cup hot water

Directions: Steep the herbs in hot water for 5-10 minutes. Strain and enjoy before bed to promote relaxation and restful sleep.

Immune-Boosting Echinacea Tincture

Ingredients:

Dried echinacea root

80-proof vodka or apple cider vinegar

Directions: Fill a glass jar halfway with echinacea root, then pour vodka or vinegar over the root until it's fully covered. Seal the jar and let it sit in a dark place for 4-6 weeks, shaking it every few days. Strain the liquid into a dark dropper bottle and take 20-30 drops daily at the first sign of illness.

Digestive Soothing Ginger Tea

Ingredients:

1 tsp freshly grated ginger

1 cup hot water

Directions: Steep the ginger in hot water for 10 minutes, strain, and sip slowly to soothe indigestion and ease nausea.

Integrating Herbal Teas and Tinctures into Daily Life

One of the best aspects of using herbal teas and tinctures is their versatility. They can be incorporated seamlessly into your day-to-day life, supporting your health in a natural and intuitive way.

Morning Ritual: Start your day with an energizing cup of peppermint or green tea or take a few drops of ashwagandha tincture to manage stress.

Midday Balance: For those hectic workdays, keep a bottle of lemon balm tincture at your desk to help ease anxiety and maintain focus.

Evening Wind-Down: Enjoy a calming tea blend of lavender, chamomile, and valerian to prepare for a restful night's sleep.

By weaving herbal teas and tinctures into your daily routine, you can create simple yet powerful wellness practices that nourish both your body and mind.

Plants have long offered us their healing gifts, and through the use of herbal teas and tinctures, we can access these gifts in a form that is easy, enjoyable, and deeply therapeutic. Whether you're sipping on a soothing tea or taking a few drops of a tincture, you are tapping into nature's most potent remedies, supporting your journey to wellness one sip at a time.

Chapter 7: Detoxing Your Body with Plants

Nature's Cleansing Allies

In today's world, our bodies are constantly exposed to toxins—from the food we eat and the air we breathe to the everyday products we use. Over time, these toxins can accumulate in our bodies, leading to sluggishness, inflammation, and other health issues. While our bodies have built-in detoxification systems (like the liver and kidneys), they sometimes need extra support to function optimally. This is where plants come in.

In this chapter, we'll explore how plant-based remedies can help cleanse and rejuvenate the body, supporting its natural detoxification processes. From liver-supporting herbs to digestive-boosting teas, you'll learn how to incorporate detoxifying plants into your daily life to enhance your overall well-being.

The Role of Plants in Detoxification

Plants have been used for centuries in traditional medicine to support the body's detoxification processes. Many plants contain phytonutrients and compounds that help cleanse the liver, kidneys, skin, and digestive system. These natural detoxifiers work by neutralizing toxins, enhancing the body's elimination processes, and protecting cells from oxidative stress.

Key Detoxifying Plants:

Milk Thistle: This herb is one of the most well-known liver detoxifiers. It contains a powerful compound called silymarin, which helps regenerate liver cells and protects them from damage caused by toxins.

Dandelion: Often considered a weed, dandelion is a potent detoxifier for both the liver and kidneys. Its diuretic properties help flush out toxins by increasing urine production, while its high antioxidant content protects cells from oxidative stress.

Turmeric: Known for its anti-inflammatory properties, curcumin (the active compound in turmeric) supports liver function by boosting the production of bile, which aids in the digestion and elimination of fats and toxins.

Cilantro: This herb is particularly effective at binding to heavy metals, such as mercury and lead, and helping the body eliminate them through the urine and digestive system.

Green Tea: Packed with antioxidants, green tea helps the body fight free radicals and supports the detoxification process. Its mild diuretic effect also helps flush out toxins through the kidneys.

Creating a Plant-Based Detox Routine

Detoxifying with plants doesn't have to be a complicated process. By making small, intentional changes to your daily routine, you can support your body's natural cleansing systems in a gentle and sustainable way.

Start Your Day with Detox Water:

Recipe: In the morning, drink a glass of warm water infused with fresh lemon juice, a few sprigs of mint, and a pinch of cayenne pepper. The lemon juice helps stimulate liver function, mint aids digestion, and cayenne pepper boosts circulation.

Sip on Herbal Teas Throughout the Day:

Drink detoxifying herbal teas such as dandelion root, ginger, and peppermint to support liver and kidney function while keeping the digestive system active. Sipping herbal tea can also help you stay hydrated, which is crucial for flushing out toxins.

Incorporate Detoxifying Foods:

Add detoxifying foods like beets, leafy greens, and cruciferous vegetables (such as broccoli and cauliflower) to your meals. These foods are rich in antioxidants and fiber, which help support liver function and aid in digestion.

Use Herbal Tinctures for Targeted Support:

For a more concentrated detox, consider using tinctures of herbs like milk thistle, burdock root, or artichoke leaf. These herbs help stimulate bile production, protect liver cells, and enhance the body's ability to eliminate waste.

The Importance of Regular Detoxification

While our bodies are designed to detoxify naturally, our modern lifestyles often overwhelm these systems. Regular detoxification can provide relief by giving your liver, kidneys, and other organs the support they need to function optimally. Some signs that you might benefit from a detox include:

Persistent fatigue

Digestive issues (such as bloating or constipation)

Skin problems (such as acne or rashes)

Brain fog or difficulty concentrating

Unexplained weight gain

By incorporating detoxifying plants into your routine, you'll help your body reset, leaving you feeling energized, clear-headed, and more in tune with your body's natural rhythms.

Developing a Detox Routine That Works for You

Detoxification is a personal journey, and it's important to listen to your body's needs. Start with small, sustainable changes, and gradually build up to more intensive detox practices as you become more comfortable. Here are a few tips for developing a detox routine that fits your lifestyle:

Begin Slowly: If you're new to detoxing, start by incorporating one or two detoxifying herbs or foods into your daily routine, such as adding a liver-supporting tea or green smoothie to your breakfast.

Stay Hydrated: Drinking plenty of water throughout the day is essential for detoxification. Water helps flush out toxins and keeps your organs functioning properly.

Monitor Your Body's Response: Pay attention to how your body reacts to detoxification practices. You might experience symptoms like headaches, fatigue, or changes in digestion as your body eliminates toxins. These are usually temporary but consult with a healthcare provider if symptoms persist.

Plants offer us a gentle, natural way to cleanse and support our bodies. By embracing their detoxifying powers, you can enhance your health and vitality in a way that feels nurturing and aligned with nature's rhythms. Whether you're sipping on herbal teas, taking a tincture, or adding detoxifying foods to your diet, remember that every small step you take brings you closer to optimal wellness.

Incorporating detoxifying plants into your daily life is not just about removing toxins—it's about fostering a deeper connection to your body and the healing gifts of nature.

Chapter 8: Strengthening Immunity with Plant Power

Nature's Defenders for a Healthier You

In a world filled with constant stressors, environmental toxins, and pathogens, maintaining a strong immune system is essential for overall health. Nature has provided us with a wealth of plants that not only nourish our bodies but also bolster our immune defenses. From immune-boosting herbs to everyday plants, integrating these natural allies into your routine can help you stay resilient in the face of illness.

In this chapter, we'll dive into the powerful relationship between plants and our immune system. You'll learn how to incorporate specific immune-boosting plants into your diet and lifestyle to help your body fend off sickness and maintain vitality.

How the Immune System Works: A Brief Overview

The immune system is our body's defense against invaders such as bacteria, viruses, and other harmful pathogens. It consists of two main components: the innate immune system (our first line of defense) and the adaptive immune system (which builds long-term immunity).

Just as we need balanced nutrition to fuel our bodies, our immune system thrives when supported by the right nutrients and compounds—many of which are found in plants. Certain plants contain phytonutrients and antioxidants that boost immune function, strengthen cells, and provide protection against inflammation.

Key Immune-Boosting Plants:

Elderberry (Sambucus nigra): Elderberries are packed with antioxidants, vitamins, and flavonoids that have been shown to boost the immune system and reduce the duration of colds and flu. The active compounds in elderberry can prevent viruses from attaching to and entering healthy cells, making it a natural defense against infections.

Echinacea (Echinacea purpurea): A well-known herb for boosting immune health, echinacea helps to stimulate the activity of white blood cells, which play a crucial role in fighting infections. It's especially effective in reducing the severity and duration of colds and flu.

Garlic (Allium sativum): This pungent kitchen staple has potent antimicrobial and antiviral properties. Garlic contains allicin, a compound that enhances immune function by stimulating the activity of white blood cells and increasing the production of immune-boosting enzymes.

Astragalus (Astragalus membranaceus): Widely used in Traditional Chinese Medicine, astragalus strengthens the immune system by increasing the body's production of immune cells and reducing inflammation. It's known for its ability to bolster resistance to colds, infections, and other illnesses.

Ginger (Zingiber officinale): Ginger's warming, anti-inflammatory properties make it an excellent ally for immune health. It's effective in combating inflammation, boosting circulation, and helping to clear respiratory pathways.

Turmeric (Curcuma longa): Turmeric is renowned for its curcumin content, which has powerful anti-inflammatory and antioxidant properties. By reducing chronic inflammation and oxidative stress, turmeric supports overall immune function and helps the body fight off infections.

Incorporating Immune-Boosting Plants into Your Daily Life

You don't need to wait until you're feeling under the weather to start incorporating immune-boosting plants into your life. By making these plants a regular part of your diet and routine, you can help strengthen your immune system and protect your body against illness all year long.

Immune-Boosting Teas:

Create a warming tea by combining fresh ginger, lemon, and honey. This blend not only soothes the throat but also provides immune-boosting properties. Ginger fights inflammation, while lemon is high in vitamin C and honey offers antimicrobial benefits.

Recipe: Elderberry Syrup. Simmer dried elderberries with cinnamon, cloves, and raw honey to create a delicious syrup that can be taken daily as an immune tonic.

Infuse Your Meals with Garlic and Turmeric:

Garlic is a versatile ingredient that can be added to soups, stews, roasted vegetables, and dressings. To maximize its immune-boosting benefits, crush fresh garlic and allow it to sit for a few minutes before cooking to release its potent compounds.

Incorporate turmeric into your diet by adding it to smoothies, soups, or golden milk. Its anti-inflammatory properties will give your immune system a daily boost.

Use Echinacea Tinctures:

Echinacea tinctures can be taken as a preventive measure or at the onset of a cold. Simply add a few drops to water or herbal tea to give your immune system an extra boost.

Astragalus Soup for Immunity:

Astragalus can be simmered in soups and broths to create an immune-boosting tonic. Add dried astragalus root to your favorite vegetable or bone broth for a nourishing and protective meal.

The Importance of a Balanced Approach

While immune-boosting plants are powerful allies, they work best when combined with a healthy lifestyle. Prioritize good nutrition, regular exercise, adequate sleep, and stress management to support your immune system holistically. A balanced approach is key to maintaining resilience and vitality.

Additionally, remember that not all immune responses are beneficial—sometimes the immune system can become overactive, leading to autoimmune issues. Therefore, always use plant remedies mindfully and in consultation with a healthcare provider, especially if you have an existing health condition.

Building Your Immune-Boosting Routine

As you begin to integrate these immune-supporting plants into your daily routine, it's important to listen to your body and adjust your practices accordingly. Here are a few tips to get started:

Consistency is Key: Incorporate immune-boosting herbs and foods regularly to keep your system strong throughout the year.

Be Mindful of Seasonal Changes: During cold and flu season, increase your intake of herbs like elderberry and echinacea to give your immune system extra support.

Know Your Body's Needs: Pay attention to how your body responds to different plants and adjust your routine as needed. Some herbs may be more beneficial for you than others, depending on your unique constitution and health concerns.

Plants have the remarkable ability to strengthen and nourish our immune system, helping us stay resilient in the face of illness and stress. By incorporating immune-boosting herbs and foods into your life, you'll not only support your physical health but also cultivate a deeper connection to the wisdom of nature.

Whether you're sipping on a warming cup of ginger tea or adding garlic to your favorite dish, these small daily practices can have a profound impact on your overall well-being. The healing power of plants is a gift from nature—embrace it, and let it guide you toward a life of vitality and wellness.

Chapter 9: Healing Skin and Body with Natural Remedies

Plant-Based Skincare for Radiance and Health

Our skin, the largest organ in our body, serves as a barrier that protects us from the outside world. It's not just an aesthetic feature—it plays a critical role in our overall health. Maintaining healthy skin goes beyond topical treatments and involves holistic care through the nourishment we provide both inside and out. Fortunately, nature has gifted us with plants that have been used for centuries to promote radiant skin, heal common issues, and protect against environmental stressors.

In this chapter, we'll explore the power of botanical skincare and natural remedies for both the skin and body. You'll learn how plant-based solutions can support your skin's vitality, offer healing properties, and bring balance to your daily skincare routine.

The Science Behind Botanical Healing for Skin

When we think about skincare, it's easy to focus on products designed to improve appearance. However, the health of our skin depends largely on how well we care for it from within. Many plant-based ingredients contain powerful antioxidants, anti-inflammatory compounds, and essential vitamins that nourish the skin at a deeper level.

Plants are rich in phytonutrients, which protect against oxidative stress caused by environmental factors like pollution, UV radiation, and toxins. These phytonutrients can slow down aging, promote cell renewal, and support the skin's natural healing process.

Antioxidants: Many plants, such as green tea, pomegranate, and berries, contain antioxidants that neutralize free radicals, reducing oxidative damage that can lead to premature aging.

Anti-inflammatory compounds: Ingredients like chamomile, calendula, and aloe vera help soothe irritated or inflamed skin, calming redness and promoting healing.

Essential oils: Certain plant-derived oils like lavender, tea tree, and rosehip contain compounds that promote hydration, reduce blemishes, and improve skin texture.

Common Plant Ingredients for Healthy Skin

The key to radiant skin often lies in simple, time-honored remedies from nature. Here are some popular plant-based ingredients you can incorporate into your skincare routine:

Aloe Vera (Aloe barbadensis): This succulent plant is renowned for its soothing, hydrating properties. Aloe vera gel contains vitamins A, C, and E, which are antioxidants that promote skin healing, reduce inflammation, and provide moisture to dry or irritated skin.

Calendula (Calendula officinalis): Known for its gentle yet powerful healing properties, calendula is a go-to herb for treating skin conditions such as eczema, rashes, and minor wounds. Its anti-inflammatory and antimicrobial properties make it ideal for soothing sensitive skin.

Lavender (Lavandula angustifolia): Lavender essential oil is beloved for its calming fragrance, but it's also an effective ingredient for skin health. It helps reduce acne, improves wound healing, and promotes relaxation, making it a popular choice for nighttime skincare routines.

Tea Tree Oil (Melaleuca alternifolia): A potent antimicrobial and anti-inflammatory oil, tea tree is often used to treat acne, fungal infections, and minor cuts. It works by reducing bacteria on the skin while calming redness and irritation.

Rosehip Oil (Rosa canina): Extracted from the seeds of wild rose bushes, rosehip oil is rich in vitamins A and C, which are crucial for skin regeneration and brightening. It's particularly effective for reducing scars, pigmentation, and fine lines.

DIY Natural Remedies for Skin and Hair

You don't need to rely on expensive skincare products to reap the benefits of plant-based healing. Here are a few simple, do-it-yourself recipes that incorporate natural ingredients to nourish and revitalize your skin and hair.

Soothing Aloe and Calendula Face Mask

Ingredients:

2 tablespoons aloe vera gel

1 teaspoon dried calendula petals (or a few drops of calendula oil)

1 teaspoon honey (optional for added hydration)

Instructions:

Mix aloe vera gel with dried calendula petals or oil in a small bowl.

Add honey for extra hydration, if desired.

Apply the mixture to your face and let it sit for 10-15 minutes.

Rinse off with warm water and pat your skin dry for a soothing, radiant glow.

Nourishing Rosehip Oil Serum

Ingredients:

1 tablespoon rosehip oil

3 drops lavender essential oil

2 drops frankincense essential oil

Instructions:

Combine all oils in a small glass bottle and shake well.

After cleansing your face, apply a few drops of the serum to your skin, focusing on areas with scars, wrinkles, or pigmentation.

Gently massage in circular motions until fully absorbed.

Tea Tree Scalp Treatment for Hair

Ingredients:

2 tablespoons coconut oil

5 drops tea tree essential oil

3 drops peppermint essential oil

Instructions:

Melt the coconut oil and mix it with tea tree and peppermint oils.

Apply the mixture directly to your scalp and massage for a few minutes to stimulate circulation and treat dandruff.

Leave on for 30 minutes or overnight before rinsing and washing your hair as usual.

The Benefits of a Plant-Based Skincare Routine

Switching to plant-based skincare isn't just about using gentler products; it's about taking a more mindful approach to self-care. Here are some benefits you'll experience when integrating plant remedies into your skincare regimen:

Reduced exposure to harmful chemicals: Many conventional skincare products contain harsh chemicals, synthetic fragrances, and preservatives that can irritate the skin. Plant-based products offer a cleaner, more natural alternative.

Supporting your skin's natural functions: Plants work in harmony with your skin's natural processes, promoting balance and healing without disrupting your body's delicate equilibrium.

Environmental sustainability: Choosing plant-based skincare is often more environmentally friendly, as many natural ingredients are sustainably sourced and biodegradable, reducing the impact on the planet.

Personal empowerment: By learning to create your own skincare remedies, you gain more control over what you're putting on your skin, tailoring products to suit your unique needs.

The Power of Consistency and Patience

While plant-based remedies can provide incredible results, it's important to remember that natural skincare often requires patience and consistency. Unlike synthetic products that offer quick fixes, plant remedies work gradually, healing the skin from within and dressing the root causes of issues.

As you integrate these plant-based solutions into your daily routine, pay attention to how your skin responds. Over time, you'll begin to see improvements in texture, tone, and overall health, revealing your skin's natural radiance.

Plants have been a source of healing and beauty for centuries, and their benefits for skin and body are as relevant today as ever. Whether you're using aloe vera to soothe sunburn or lavender to calm your mind before bed, these natural remedies offer a holistic approach to skincare that goes beyond surface-level beauty. By embracing plant-based healing, you nurture not only your skin but your entire well-being.

Your skin, like the rest of your body, deserves to be treated with the gentleness and care that nature provides.

Chapter 10: The Future of Plant-Based Medicine

Exploring the New Horizons in Natural Healing

As we look toward the future of healthcare and wellness, one thing is becoming increasingly clear: plant-based medicine is here to stay. From ancient remedies that have stood the test of time to cutting-edge scientific research on the therapeutic properties of plants, nature's medicine cabinet continues to offer exciting possibilities for enhancing human health.

This chapter delves into the future of plant-based medicine, exploring the trends, advancements, and innovations that are reshaping the landscape of natural healing. We will consider how science and technology are expanding our understanding of plant compounds and their healing potential. Furthermore, we'll explore the increasing role that plants will play in modern medicine, preventative care, and holistic well-being.

The Evolution of Plant-Based Therapies

In recent years, there has been a surge of interest in plant-based therapies. While herbal remedies and medicinal plants have been used for centuries in traditional healing practices, modern science is now catching up, validating the benefits of many natural treatments through rigorous research.

Key trends in plant-based medicine include:

Scientific Validation: Researchers around the world are investigating the bioactive compounds in plants and their therapeutic effects. For instance, studies on cannabidiol (CBD), a compound derived from cannabis, have demonstrated its potential to alleviate pain, reduce inflammation, and help manage anxiety.

Phytotherapy in Mainstream Healthcare: Phytotherapy, the use of plant extracts for medicinal purposes, is no longer confined to alternative medicine. Physicians are increasingly integrating herbal remedies into conventional treatments, particularly for conditions like inflammation, digestive disorders, and mental health concerns.

Personalized Plant-Based Medicine: Advances in genetic research are opening doors to personalized medicine, where an individual's genetic makeup can inform which plant-based remedies might be most effective. This customized approach could revolutionize how we use plants for healing, offering more targeted and efficient treatments.

Harnessing the Power of Plant Compounds with Technology

As technology continues to advance, so too does our ability to unlock the full healing potential of plants. From sophisticated extraction methods to digital tools that enhance our understanding of plant biology, innovation is driving new possibilities for plant-based medicine.

Advanced Extraction Techniques

Traditional methods of preparing plant-based remedies, such as infusions and decoctions, are giving way to more advanced extraction techniques. New technologies allow scientists to isolate specific bioactive compounds with greater precision, resulting in more potent and consistent products.

Supercritical CO2 extraction, for example, is a process that uses carbon dioxide at high pressure and low temperature to extract plant compounds without the need for harmful solvents. This method is widely used in the production of essential oils and herbal extracts, preserving the plant's natural integrity while maximizing its therapeutic benefits.

Biotechnology and Genetic Engineering

Biotechnology is revolutionizing plant-based medicine by enabling scientists to enhance the potency and efficacy of medicinal plants. Through genetic engineering, researchers can increase the concentration of beneficial compounds in plants or even transfer healing properties from one species to another.

In addition, the use of plant stem cells in cosmetics and skincare products is a growing trend. These stem cells are rich in antioxidants and growth factors, making them highly effective in promoting skin regeneration and reducing signs of aging.

Plant-Based Solutions for Chronic Diseases

One of the most exciting areas of research in plant-based medicine is its potential to combat chronic diseases, which are responsible for a significant portion of global healthcare costs. Plants offer a wide range of bioactive compounds that can help address the root causes of chronic illnesses such as cardiovascular disease, diabetes, and cancer.

Cardiovascular Health

Many plants are rich in compounds that support heart health. For example, flavonoids found in berries, citrus fruits, and dark chocolate have been shown to improve blood vessel function, reduce blood pressure, and lower the risk of heart disease.

Hawthorn (Crataegus spp.), a plant traditionally used in European herbal medicine, has gained recognition for its ability to strengthen the heart muscle, improve circulation, and reduce symptoms of heart failure.

Diabetes Management

Several plants have shown promise in helping manage blood sugar levels and reduce the risk of type 2 diabetes. For instance, berberine, an alkaloid found in plants like goldenseal and barberry, has been studied for its ability to regulate blood glucose and improve insulin sensitivity.

Fenugreek seeds are also well-known for their blood sugar-lowering effects, making them a valuable addition to a diabetes management plan.

Cancer Prevention and Treatment

Research into the anticancer properties of plants is growing, with many promising results. Curcumin, the active compound in turmeric, has demonstrated the ability to inhibit the growth of cancer cells and reduce inflammation, a key factor in the development of cancer.

Green tea extract, rich in polyphenols such as epigallocatechin gallate (EGCG), has been shown to slow the progression of certain cancers by preventing cell mutations and inhibiting tumor growth.

The Future of Plant-Based Medicine in Healthcare

As plant-based therapies continue to evolve, their integration into mainstream healthcare is poised to increase. Here are some ways plant medicine may shape the future of healthcare:

Preventative Medicine

In the future, we may see a stronger emphasis on preventative care, with plant-based therapies playing a key role. Herbal supplements, dietary interventions, and natural therapies will likely be used more widely to prevent illness and support overall well-being before pharmaceutical interventions become necessary.

Holistic Health Practices

As more people seek out natural, holistic approaches to health, the demand for integrative healthcare models that incorporate both conventional medicine and plant-based treatments will grow. Hospitals, clinics, and wellness centers may increasingly offer holistic care options, including phytotherapy, acupuncture, and nutritional counseling.

Education and Accessibility

One challenge that remains in the field of plant-based medicine is accessibility. Not everyone has the knowledge or resources to incorporate plant therapies into their health routines. The future may bring more widespread education about the benefits of medicinal plants, along with increased accessibility through online platforms, community workshops, and affordable herbal products.

The future of plant-based medicine is bright, with boundless possibilities for improving health, preventing disease, and enhancing overall well-being. As we continue to explore the therapeutic power of plants, we are not only reconnecting with ancient healing traditions but also forging new pathways to a healthier, more balanced future.

Our journey with plant-based medicine is just beginning, and the future holds exciting prospects for both individuals and healthcare systems worldwide. Embrace the possibilities and continue to explore the healing power of nature.

Chapter 11: Healing Skin and Body with Natural Remedies

Embracing the Power of Botanicals for Radiant Health

The skin, the body's largest organ, is not only our first line of defense against the elements but also a reflection of our overall health and well-being. When nourished properly, it can glow with vitality and resilience, but neglect or exposure to harmful substances can lead to dryness, inflammation, and premature aging.

In this chapter, we will explore the remarkable power of plant-based remedies to heal, rejuvenate, and protect both the skin and the body. From soothing sunburns with aloe vera to reducing inflammation with chamomile, plants offer an abundance of natural solutions for skincare and holistic health. We will dive deep into the science behind botanical ingredients and discover how they work to promote healing, restore balance, and enhance the skin's natural radiance.

The Science Behind Plant-Based Skincare

Modern skincare is evolving beyond chemical-laden products, with many people turning to the plant world for natural alternatives. Unlike synthetic ingredients, plant-based remedies offer gentle yet potent healing effects without the harsh side effects. Plants are packed with vitamins, antioxidants, and anti-inflammatory compounds that nourish the skin, repair damage, and protect against environmental stressors.

Antioxidant-Rich Botanicals

Antioxidants are nature's defense mechanism against oxidative stress, which is one of the primary causes of skin aging. Plants like green tea, rosemary, and rosehip contain high levels of antioxidants that can neutralize free radicals, protecting the skin from damage caused by pollution, UV radiation, and stress.

Green tea extract, for instance, is rich in polyphenols, which help reduce inflammation, protect the skin from sun damage, and promote a more even complexion.

Rosehip oil, a popular anti-aging remedy, is packed with vitamins A and C, which are essential for collagen production and skin regeneration.

Hydration and Moisture Locking

Moisture is key to maintaining youthful, supple skin, and plants offer some of the best sources of hydration. Ingredients like aloe vera, cucumber extract, and hyaluronic acid (derived from plants) have become skincare staples for their ability to lock in moisture and plump the skin.

Aloe vera: Known for its soothing properties, aloe vera not only hydrates but also calms irritated skin, making it a perfect remedy for sunburns, eczema, and other inflammatory skin conditions.

Cucumber extract: Rich in water and vitamins, cucumber helps to cool, refresh, and hydrate the skin, reducing puffiness and promoting a more youthful appearance.

Anti-Inflammatory and Healing Properties

Inflammation is at the root of many skin conditions, from acne to dermatitis. Plants like chamomile, calendula, and lavender are revered for their anti-inflammatory and calming effects, helping to soothe redness, swelling, and irritation.

Chamomile extract: With its gentle, soothing properties, chamomile is ideal for sensitive skin and can help to calm conditions like rosacea and eczema.

Calendula oil: Derived from marigold flowers, calendula is a powerful healing agent that can speed up the recovery of wounds, reduce scarring, and calm inflamed skin.

DIY Natural Remedies for Healthy Skin

While store-bought products can be effective, creating your own natural skincare remedies allows you to take full control of the ingredients you're using. By using fresh, organic ingredients, you can customize treatments to suit your specific skin type and concerns. Here are a few simple DIY remedies to try at home:

Aloe Vera and Honey Soothing Mask

Aloe vera is renowned for its healing properties, while honey is a natural humectant, meaning it draws moisture into the skin.

Ingredients:

2 tablespoons of fresh aloe vera gel

1 tablespoon of raw honey

Instructions:

Mix the aloe vera gel and honey until well-blended.

Apply the mixture to clean skin and leave it on for 15-20 minutes.

Rinse off with warm water and follow up with a gentle moisturizer.

This mask is perfect for calming irritated skin, reducing redness, and giving your complexion a hydration boost.

Green Tea and Cucumber Toner

Green tea and cucumber are both packed with antioxidants and soothing properties, making this toner perfect for revitalizing tired skin.

Ingredients:

1 cup brewed green tea (cooled)

½ cucumber, pureed

Instructions:

Brew a cup of green tea and allow it to cool.

Blend the cucumber into a puree and mix it with the green tea.

Strain the mixture to remove any large particles, then transfer it to a spray bottle.

Use this toner after cleansing to refresh the skin and tighten pores.

Herbal Oils for Skin Rejuvenation

Essential oils and carrier oils, extracted from plants, offer another layer of benefits for the skin. These oils are rich in vitamins, fatty acids, and antioxidants, making them invaluable for hydration, healing, and anti-aging.

Rosehip Seed Oil

Rosehip seed oil is a powerhouse of nutrients, including vitamins A and C, essential fatty acids, and antioxidants. It's particularly effective for reducing the appearance of scars, fine lines, and hyperpigmentation.

Usage: Massage a few drops of rosehip oil into your skin before bed, allowing it to penetrate and rejuvenate overnight.

Jojoba Oil

Jojoba oil is unique because its structure closely resembles the skin's natural sebum. This means it's easily absorbed and helps to regulate oil production, making it ideal for both dry and oily skin types.

Usage: Apply jojoba oil as a lightweight moisturizer after cleansing or use it as a makeup remover.

Common Plant Ingredients in Skincare and Their Benefits

Plants offer a diverse range of compounds that can benefit the skin in countless ways. Here are some common plant ingredients you'll find in natural skincare products and their associated benefits:

Tea tree oil: Known for its antimicrobial properties, tea tree oil is excellent for treating acne and preventing infections.

Lavender: This calming plant not only promotes relaxation but also helps to soothe irritated skin and accelerate wound healing.

Shea butter: Extracted from the nuts of the shea tree, this rich butter is packed with vitamins and fatty acids that deeply moisturize and nourish the skin.

Witch hazel: A natural astringent, witch hazel helps to tighten pores, reduce oiliness, and calm inflammation.

Healing the Body with Plant-Based Remedies

While skincare is important, plants can also support the healing and rejuvenation of the body as a whole. From muscle soreness to digestive issues, natural remedies offer gentle, effective solutions for common ailments.

Soothing Muscle Soreness

After a long day or an intense workout, muscle soreness can leave you feeling fatigued. Plants like arnica, peppermint, and eucalyptus are known for their ability to reduce inflammation and ease pain

Arnica gel: Applied topically, arnica gel can help to reduce bruising and soothe sore muscles.

Digestive Support

Herbal remedies can also aid in digestion, promoting a healthy gut and relieving discomfort. Herbs like ginger, fennel, and peppermint have been used for centuries to ease indigestion, bloating, and nausea.

Ginger tea: Drinking ginger tea after a meal can stimulate digestion and reduce nausea, making it an excellent remedy for digestive upset.

The future of skincare and body care lies in returning to nature's roots. By embracing plant-based remedies, we can nourish our skin and body with the healing power of botanicals, creating routines that enhance both our outer radiance and inner well-being.

Chapter 12: Reflections

Cultivating Wellness with Nature's Gifts

As we bring *The Plant Prescription* to a close, I encourage you to carry the wisdom of nature's remedies with you, using them not only as tools for healing but as pathways to a more balanced and vibrant life. Just as the plants we've explored in this book grow with patience and care, so too does your well-being thrive when nurtured with intention and love.

Each herb, root, and leaf you've learned about is a reminder that nature has long provided us with everything we need to restore balance, foster resilience, and strengthen our connection to the world around us. Whether you're sipping a calming tea, incorporating an herbal remedy into your routine, or simply spending time with plants, remember that wellness is not a destination, but an ongoing journey of harmony between body, mind, and spirit.

By embracing plant-based healing, you're not only taking steps toward physical health, but also opening yourself to a deeper connection with the natural world. This is an invitation to continue exploring the gentle power of nature's pharmacy and to cultivate a life filled with vitality and peace.

Further Explorations

If you've enjoyed discovering the healing potential of plants in *The Plant Prescription*, I invite you to explore my other books. In *Rooted in Calm*, we delve into how plants can help us manage stress and foster inner peace, while *Blooming Minds* explores how plants can inspire creativity and mental clarity.

May these books continue to guide you on your path of wellness, creativity, and connection to the world around you.

Remember: The seeds of well-being are within you. With the nurturing power of plants, you have the tools to cultivate a life of health, balance, and harmony. Keep tending to your wellness and let nature's gifts continue to enrich your journey.

About the Author

Aspen Sunhaven's lifelong love affair with nature began in the sun-dappled forests and wildflower meadows of her childhood. Exploring these natural havens instilled in her a deep appreciation for the intricate beauty and quiet resilience of plants, and a profound understanding of the interconnectedness of all living things.

Driven by a desire to share her passion and inspire others, Aspen's writing weaves together personal experiences, scientific insights, and practical wisdom. She believes that cultivating a connection with plants can enrich our lives in countless ways - from fostering a sense of wonder and inner peace to promoting sustainable living and a deeper appreciation for the natural world.

When she's not writing, you'll find Aspen tending her own flourishing garden, exploring nearby trails, or curled up with a beloved book and a steaming cup of tea. Her greatest hope is that her work will spark curiosity, ignite a passion for nature, and encourage readers to embark on their own transformative journeys of discovery.